CHAPTER 1

INTRODUCTION

Erotic or sensual massage is one of the best ways to exchange all the love that there can be in a couple. This sensual massage is mainly used to stimulate or exalt the libido of the man or the woman to be more in harmony with the desires of his or her spouse.

It could enter the range of foreplay, thus contributing to the increase in sensitivity and the receptivity of the senses.

The erotic massage is, paradoxically, often practiced by professional masseuses naked. It contributes against all the odds to help men who have problems of premature ejaculation through a wider distribution of sexual energies too often concentrated on particular points.

Erotic massage does not translate as "sexual massage". This type of massage, sensual by definition, is often accompanied by massage oils, if possible hypoallergenic.

The principle is very simple: coat the body of your partner with oils and either practice mutual or

Erotic Massage for Couples

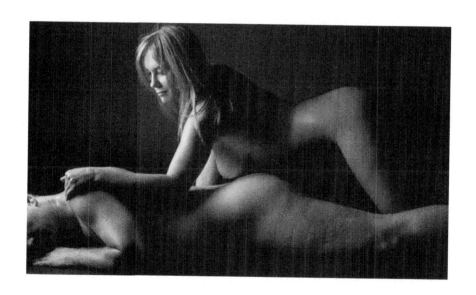

Table of Contents

alternating massage, or one of the two accomplices is devoted to the other, alternatively what is also an approach sensual, or the two bodies gently rub against each other. This hyper-sensory exchange allows the massed person to feel intense emotions, putting him in a state of receptivity, awakening the senses to well-being.

The most crucial step of the erotic massage allows spreading throughout the body the eroticism, the sensuality generated by the previous movements so that the ultimate enjoyment is tasted by the whole body and not only (as produced so often in "ordinary" love relationships) by the genitals.

History of Erotic Massage

You may ask where this erotic massage came from. Yes, this is a good question, but the answer may be difficult to give with exactitude, for the simple reason that the erotic massage is mostly appealing to the touch, the origins of the real erotic massage can be varied!

The notion of pleasure associated with touch comes first of all from the cradle when our mother caresses us and transmits all her love to us by her touch, the feel of her hug and her kiss, but this is not at all erotic.

Only, if we go back more in time, the erotic massage would have known its beginnings in Asia with the link between the mind and the body and all the Buddhist culture. By the way, what is paradoxical today is that Countries like Thailand, more precisely Bangkok, are the realm of this erotic massage, a concept that moves away from the purity of Buddhism.

Among others, when Vatsyayana wrote the Kama Sutra in India in the eighth century, he was preparing for future generations a real work of philosophy, psychology, Hindu teachings and a classic guide of sexual sensuality, reflecting the social and sexual customs of his time.

The teachings of the Kama Sutra include the use of oils, perfumes, and erotic massages to increase the senses and sexual pleasure ("Kama" being the name of the Hindu God of love and "Sutra" meaning manual or guide).

Other thinkers say that the exact origin of erotic massage is in the time of the Romans where sexual orgies allowed touching and massaging almost everything that moved in the human body mass naked and voluptuous for sex!

Buttocks massage, Kamasutra, Massage of the genitals of a man, in any case, the touch is a very often neglected aspect in our modern daily life. Which means that many people still do not know what an erotic massage is either for lack of knowledge or misplaced taboo fueled by both our old Catholic roots and by the widespread belief that erotic massage goes with unhealthy and depraved sexual life.

We live in a society where everything is and must be ultra-fast that we do not even take the time to touch and soak up the heat of our partner apart from the purely sexual act!

The erotic massage divides several distinct parts but intimately connected. First, you have to start with the full massage, concerning all parts of the body. The goal of this step is relaxation. This type of massage is found in many books that are currently on the market. Then, the second step consists of a series of caresses, or movements, covering the whole body. This section is linked with the one that is more interested in the erogenous zones of your partner's body, but, as much as possible, avoiding an over-excitation of the genital areas.

Erotic massage has several interdependent components.

Again, there is no need to go through the steps, and you spoil the "sauce". Admit from the outset that these steps must be followed to the letter, that this approach is essential to the success of the erotic massage.

Once this is admitted, you will see that everything is going according to plan, and the desired effects will occur as desired. So, take advantage of this erotic massage guide to make up for lost time with your current or future partner!

CHAPTER 2. SEXUAL PSYCHOLOGY OF COUPLES THAT LIVE TOGETHER FOR A LONG TIME

Most couples that live together for a long time love each other but tend not to make love anymore. Some couples continue to love each other despite the absence of sex. They say the marriage does not suffer because of lack of sex. How do they keep the flame when the desire is gone?

Some couples do not even remember the last time they made love. There is a story of a couple in my neighborhood, Mathew and Eva, around 48 years of age, married for 21 years, happy parents of two children. They have, by their admission, gradually put aside their sexuality. This does not prevent them from laughing together, handing each other out on the street or sleeping against each other.

Without claiming it or being part of the 'no sex' movement in recent years, Mathew and Eva have found a marital balance that belongs to them, refusing to make this lack of frolics a "problem". A choice assumed less rare than it seems, the heart has its reasons that sometimes the body ignores. Now someone may ask, love without making love, is it possible? How is sexual desire born? What is the physical desire for men and women?

Often, it is after giving birth, the loss of a loved one or a job, mourning situations that slumber the libido (sexual drive) and, in the case of unemployment, bear a blow to the esteem of self, that the couple interrupts all sexual activity. Hugs become scarce until they disappear entirely from the marital landscape. Because the less we make love, the less the desire is there, since the sexual drive is self-powered, more like a battery. Our partner excites our desire not just because he/she is beautiful or handsome, feels good and is intelligent, but because it occupies a special place in our psychic organization.

According to Freudian theory, unconsciously, a woman often sees in her partner the man who will make her a mother or a savior who has symbolically killed her innocence to free her from being a little girl. A man tends to see in his companion, which will allow him to overcome his father. This is why the birth of a child who is known to be the last of the siblings sometimes augurs a long period without sex or marks outright the end of lovemaking.

Therefore, spouses must invent another sexuality. Hence the issues of motherhood and paternity have disappeared. This is also the case at menopause. They have to reconstruct inner scenarios, this time focusing mainly on enjoyment alone and challenging psychic task if their relationship to pleasure is tinged with guilt.

The absence of sex is not painful in itself. It is the frustration, the impossibility of accessing the desired pleasure, which makes you sick. Freud, the inventor of a theory linking sexuality and neurosis, had ceased all sexual life in his forties.

A reality which reminds us that, for psychoanalysis, in this matter, precisely, there is no norm. "Love comes in many forms, and it is possible to find other ways to cement a couple. I would even say that when we stay together despite abstinence, it is probably because of love, because we decide to invest in our family, in common interests, in the comfort of life together. "

According to most couples, physical distance does not happen overnight. Most women always say that it is after their last delivery, that the pace of lovemaking begins to get dull. "Not only did I fail to enjoy, but I was in pain. Mathew ended up being afraid of making me suffer, said Eva. So he stopped asking me. At first, I was afraid that he wanted to go elsewhere, but I ended up believing him when he assured me that it did not matter much considering the love we have. "

"It is not a philosophy of life or a bias, says Mathew. If the circumstances had been different, if we had not encountered these difficulties after the birth of our daughter, perhaps we would have a more sexual relationship today. I did not make a cross on this aspect of our relationship, but today, it is so. Moreover, curiously, I have the feeling that we have developed a different sensuality, which is expressed, for example in the way we enjoy a good wine together or a meal in our favorite restaurant. What counts above all is the desire we feel to be together, and this desire is always strong. "

Sex is a matter of impulses, but they find themselves satisfied in various ways. The pleasures of the mouth - to taste a good wine, to share an excellent dinner - satisfy the oral impulse. To visit an exhibition, to watch a film, to travel, to discover new landscapes satisfy the requirements of the sexual drive - the drive of the gaze. It should not be thought that these activities are only pale and weak substitutes for genital sexuality, which would be the royal voice to pleasure. It is the sexual drive that, sublimated, that is to say, deviated from its primary purpose, inspires artists, makes them creative.

Open to sensuality and feel better touch, love. We confuse sensuality and sexual pleasure, "sensoriality" and animality. However, there are ways to reconnect to the world. This reconciliation is essential: it is about our joy of living!

We must distinguish between sensuality and sexuality. I see couples who do not make love in the academic sense of the word, but who continue to kiss, to touch, to cuddle — so many proofs of love. By definition, I receive in my office only couples who want to get out of this abstinence. However, I am often amazed at the time they have been able to spend without suffering in their marriages.

The desire and the sharing are two essential elements to the longevity of a couple. When the sexual activity diminishes or even disappears, what keeps love is the ability to have fun together. Two people who continue to love each other without sexual relationships have generally been able to identify what feeds them personally. There is a flow of love between the partners, but not necessarily in a sexual form. To reduce love to sexuality would not do honor to the infinite ways by which one can manifest one's feelings to another.

"There is so much tenderness between us". Jane and Eric, young retirees in DC, have also seen their desire dull over the years. "Eric has never been a lightning bolt, and I am probably a generation of women who have not learned to talk about these things. Initially, I suffered from the situation, and I thought that I did not attract him anymore, that he had met someone else. However, he swore to me that no, that he loved only me; only that the sex aspect did not work too well. Sometimes I tell myself that we should have talked to a doctor, see if there was a solution, but today is a bit late, and it has become a little taboo. ", she said.

Moreover, if there were a way to revive the flame, would she? "Not necessarily," answered Jane. Our agreement is lovely, and there is so much tenderness between us that I would be afraid to nudge all that. "A confession that is not very surprising. When a couple is delighted with abstinence, it is usually because, for one or the other, or both, sexuality refers to suffering, whether it is a physiological dysfunction or a childhood injury. Awakening desire also involves awakening this suffering, whatever it may be. "

There is indeed an aggressive, animal component in the sexual drive that can scare you away. Some people who do not feel good enough or lack self-esteem are unable to associate sex with feeling as if the materiality of the flesh is against the purity of love. Also, they will choose to take refuge in a bond of tenderness instead of the reassuring cocoon. No pathology in this decision, since it allows a development.

If Mathew and Eva or Jane and Eric live serenely, this love becomes platonic, and it is above all because everyone seems to have accepted, and no one feels any form of frustration. Because, as soon as one of the partners no longer finds his or her balance, the beautiful tenderness that seemed to last for centuries falters. It can sometimes take months, if not years, without any sexual activity. Moreover, then, one day, what seemed to suit both is no longer satisfactory. At that time, we must act to save the couple. Otherwise, the person who no longer supports the situation will decide to go elsewhere.

To stay together, although one does not make love anymore, supposes, in fact, a common definition of what the couple is: two beings who support each other, two halves finally united, a society of mutual admiration? We all dream - or almost - of total complicity linking eroticism and intellectual understanding harmoniously. However, with the years, the bodies change the sexual tastes too. Also, the fantasies of both partners will not necessarily evolve at the same pace.

Also, an association constituted mainly based on shared passions; the same ideological or philosophical commitments are more likely to resist the time that a couple created due to an irresistible sexual attraction. Less exciting at first glance, but is it so safe?

CHAPTER 3. TYPES OF EROTIC MASSAGE

Each massage has its specificity. Some bring only pleasure to the body, and others help you relax, some even palliate various disorders or pathologies. So you understand, we do not use the massage to feel good, but also to heal. Moreover, the types of massage that we are going to introduce are some of the most successful ones!

Californian massage to relax and fight various tensions

It is in the Californian massage that one finds the use of oils and essential oils. This is the most widespread and popular type of massage in the world. It targets two kinds of well-being. On the one hand, it relieves the body of various tensions occurring in the muscles and gives you physical well-being. On the other hand, it soothes mental tensions and thus brings mental well-being. This type of massage, therefore, deals with the body and the mind at the same time.

The Californian massage works by relaxing the patient, soothing his pain, and awakening his body-mind awareness. It directly attacks the tensions felt by the body and mind of the person being massaged. These tensions are released, thanks to the gentle and fluid movements performed by the masseur or the massage therapist. These movements consist of effleurages: the massage therapist touches the skin and then specifies its actions so that the tensions are lightened. This precision will also lead to the awakening of the memory of the person being massaged so that it determines the origin of his stress, which facilitates the therapy by the Californian massage.

Note that the latter is used to treat chronic disorders, pain in the muscles, joints, and many others. Californian massage is categorized as one of the most relaxing massages, suitable for people who continually stress or feel various tensions in their body. However, beware, there are some mistakes not to make in other to make an excellent relaxing massage.

Reflexology, to fight against stress and anxiety

Reflexology is the massage that fights anxiety and stress while relaxing the person massaged for a long time. It is real therapy to fight different diseases in the body. It eliminates toxins in the body and relieves the liver, heart, stomach, and many body parts prone to disorders. It even restores the blood flow. It targets reflex points on the body, such as feet, hands, or ears. The masseur presses on these zones by exerting an absolute pressure.

Ayurvedic massage to regain your body balance

Ayurveda massage is native to India, specifically from the region of Ayurveda. It consists of a stimulation of the seven chakras and uses, for this purpose, hot oil. The masseur applies it on the body of the person being massaged or on his forehead and presses different Ayurvedic points so that the equilibrium is restored. It rebalances the body and gives it, at the same time, energy. Thus, the masseur practices it in the greatest tranquility, very gently. It mostly massages the back that the Indians call "sacred zone" of the body. Because it relaxes the person massaged, it is therefore advisable to the eternal stressed and those who have back pain.

The amma massage, to relax very quickly

One of the characteristics of the amma massage is its particularly short duration. In this sense, it is mostly seated, but some people prefer to apply it by extending their massage. Amma massage is an alloy of traditional medicines from China and Japan. It provides energy and serenity to the person being massaged because the massager manipulates various points which are on the joints or the muscles.

Because it can be practiced while sitting, the amma massage can be done almost anywhere, provided that you can stall a massage chair. It is ideal for modest as it does not require undressing. It is done in a quarter of an hour and allows you to relax very quickly. This is best appreciated by the most eager and those who have no time to lose.

Shiatsu massage, to rebalance the body

The term shiatsu means "finger pressure". Shiatsu massage, therefore, consists of finger pressure on specific parts of the body. This type of massage is from China but has been revisited by the Japanese. It intervenes by rebalancing the circulation of energy in the body. To do this, the masseur presses pressure zones. These lead to the energy flow of the body. They are identified beforehand by the masseur.

Shiatsu massage is a massage that ends rather quickly and that one practice dressed. If you experience temporary fatigue, have insomnia or are stressed continuously, shiatsu massage is right for you.

Thai massage, to say goodbye to chronic fatigue

Among the many massages that are listed, Thai massage is mainly known for reducing or even wiping out fatigue. It is practiced on a futon laid on the floor and with the help of many massage oils. It is done in several movements as rhythmic as fast. It delivers the receiver of his/her negative emotions and allows him/her to find the balance of his/her body.

The masseur practices it by stretching, twisting, and kneading the area to be massaged, which is why Thai massage is a bit painful or a bit tiring. Rest assured, fatigue and pain disappear the next day, and your body will feel crazy well-being!

For the smooth running and the effectiveness of your massage, know that there are mistakes not to commit during a massage. They mainly concern the amateurs and are summarized not to touch or to massage in a very delicate way the neck and the abdomen. Sensitive areas such as the armpits, they are downright avoided!

Hot stones

The hot stone massage is very gentle and soothing. You will be massaged with warm basalt stones coated with essential oils on strategic points of your body, for a very relaxing effect.

CHAPTER 4. BEGINNERS' SECRETS TO THEIR FIRST EROTIC MASSAGE

To make an excellent erotic massage, there are, of course, rules to respect, especially for beginners. Here they are;

• Be clean: make sure you are both clean. Hygiene is essential in general and especially for a massage. You could even take a shower for two before starting the massage but, avoid making love in the shower before the naughty massage. Make the pleasure last for more enjoyment during and after the erotic massage.

• Prepare the atmosphere: it must make a pleasant temperature in the room to not be cold and risk keeping the muscles contracted. Being nude, you must feel comfortable and not having in mind to slip under a blanket...

• Adapt the room: choose a room or any other place that is best for relaxation. Soft light, background music, candles, and cell phones off.

• Choose the comfort: whether you choose the floor, the bed or the sofa, it must be comfortable for both of you. Do not hesitate to put cushions and soft and fluffy materials.

• Select oils: For your erotic massage, you will need to select the appropriate massage oils. You can even agree on one or more scents that appeal to you. The smell must please both of you. I recommend organic vegetable oil.

• Eat light before the massage: avoid a heavy meal before the naughty massage. You may end up on sex games, and you will certainly make love so better to feel comfortable. You risk ruining everything with a full stomach or bloated.

• Remove jewelry: nothing more unpleasant than a massage made with jewelry. So we remove them! It will be more pleasant for the one who massages and also for the one who receives the massage. It also limits the risk of injury.

• Keep a hand on your body: during a massage, you should always keep at least one hand on your body so as not to cut the sexual contact. It is very important. You must continuously be in contact with each other.

• Listening to each other: during an erotic massage, you have to be attentive to the other person. Thus, you will have to adapt the pressure of your movements according to the reactions of your partner. You will also have to pay attention to the places in her body that seem to do her more or less well. Also, pay attention to his breathing which will tell you if what you are doing is pleasant or very unpleasant.

• Vary the techniques: do not always do the same thing in the same places. You must vary the methods between kneading, effleurage, kneading, and many others. Avoid painful areas if, for example, there are bruises. Do not forget that the goal of erotic massage is to provide pleasure but also and above all to listen to your partner and his/her pleasures.

• Reverse the roles: it does not always have to be one of the partners that massages the other. Of course, if you decide whom to mass and who gets massaged, go to the end and enjoy both fully.

On the other hand, also reverse the roles for even more pleasure and spice.

• Let it go: the erotic massage must allow you to let go completely, both of you. Add kisses and tender gestures to your massage for even more sensuality and complicity.

So much for the basic rules to follow for an excellent erotic massage. Remember that the secret of a good erotic massage is to listen to each other.

One last thing: the massaged partner will necessarily be naked. For the partner who massages, agree to wear a sexy outfit or lingerie or to be naked too. It is up to you to see what makes you feel good and excites you the most.

You must both enjoy this sensual and erotic experience. However, know that your both bodies must be in contact, so better to have the least fabric possible between you two.

Things You Need for Your First Erotic Massage

To carry out an erotic massage, you have to know how to choose the right equipment. A bed or a massage table is, for example, far from ideal to highlight sensuality in all its forms. Indeed, this furniture is not suitable because it is too high for a real sensual massage between two completely naked bodies. The idea is to practice erotic massage on a mattress that will be installed directly on the floor.

For optimal comfort, include plaids, blankets, bath towels, cushions, a mattress. You will have chosen flexible clothes that allow you to move freely, fluids, and ease in your movements.

ACCESSORIES FOR AN EROTIC MASSAGE

It is better to choose massage oil for two. If you have chosen coconut oil, for example, it would be a shame to learn at the beginning that your partner has a deep dislike for its oily texture.

For an erotic massage, you would prefer a dry oil that the skin absorbs quickly. Argan oil is a good base. Its light scent and its many virtues make it ideal for this type of massage. You can add, according to your preferences, an essential oil: jasmine (subtly aphrodisiac), rose or more masculine perfumes such as patchouli, cedarwood, and ylang-ylang. Check that these essential oils are well suited for massages. Sandalwood oil and sweet almond oil give a blend ideally suited to a foot massage.

CHAPTER 5. 25 TOP RATED SENSUAL MASSAGE TIPS

Providing unique sensations to a person is not given to everyone, and only concerns those who master the techniques of the erotic massage, a massage that emphasizes the sensual connotation. It is a technique that takes the mass in another dimension where sensuality makes sense. It is a discipline open to all to allow relaxing in another way and get rid of stress completely.

No one should do erotic massage because this discipline requires the mastery of specific techniques. An inexperienced person in this area will certainly not increase the excitement of the massed. The goal with the erotic massage is to raise the excitement with different phases while remaining in the emotional side of the massage.

Creating an atmosphere is one of the main goals of a professional masseuse. You play with your partner's hands and his/her body to make reign a purely sensual environment. This atmosphere must go hand in hand with an atmosphere that is both calm and relaxing. That is why most experienced masseuses always opt for dim light, for example, by placing candles in the room. Without forgetting the soft music, they make sure that the ambient temperature can offer a warm and soothing atmosphere.

BELOW ARE 25 TIPS FOR AN EXCELLENT SENSUAL MASSAGE;

Our body presents different erogenous zones. We can start with the legs and feet. A foot massage can be both soothing and exciting. It can spread chills all over the body and produce a great feeling of pleasure. Reflexology teaches us that different organs are connected to certain areas of the feet.

Your partner is lying on his/her back. The atmosphere is relaxed. You took care to place a small cushion under his/her knees. Sitting at their feet, you heat the oil in your hands.

1. Choose a quiet place at home. Make sure you are not disturbed by anyone.

2. Take his feet gently and delicately, then start to massage. Take the left foot and practice circular movements around the bony structures of the ankle (malleolus) in a clockwise direction. Do the same for the right foot.

3. With the tips of the first three fingers of both hands, make circular movements around the outer bone structure. Five circles in one direction and then years in the other. Perform these movements in the shape of eight, slowly. Vary the weight of the pressures and the amplitude of the gestures.

4. You can talk to your partner and questioning him about his feelings. One attention + another = love gain for your partner.

5. Take the left foot of your partner. Remember to cover his right foot to keep him warm.

6. Put oil on the kick and the plant. Make it penetrate up from the middle of the foot to the ankle, from one hand to another.

7. The foot placed between your palms, slide your hands with a single gesture towards the toes. Repeat several times.

8. The kick in both hands, slide them slowly on each side up to the toes.

9. Run the soles of your foot with your fingertips, exerting light pressure. Reassemble to the ankle. Perform this movement several times.

10. Find out about your partner's feelings.

11. Using your two thumbs, stroke the kick. Perform gentle movements around the ankle.

12. Hold your foot with your left hand. Apply slight pressure to the center of the plant with your right thumb while drawing circles.

13. Go to the toes. Grab each of them with your thumb, forefinger and middle finger for gentle kisses.

14. Cover the left foot and take care of your right foot in the same way.

15. Cover both of your partner's feet. Add oil on top and plant. Caress the external malleolus forming the figure of eight.

16. Take both of his heels in your hands, and swing his legs, pulling his feet towards you.

17. The massage is practiced naked or partially undressed, and the room must be well heated.

18. Create a soothing, warm, and subdued atmosphere.

19. Perfume the space with essential oils of your choice.

20. Add some candles and spread some soft music.

21. No rush. Everything is done slowly and gently.

22. Practice different touches on the seven chakras, i.e., the energy points of the body.

23. Combine kneading, light pressure and effleurage movements slowly and gently.

24. Your hands roam and wrap your partner's body from head to toe (sense of circulation of sexual energy), producing a sense of sensations that wakes him up, thrilling and thrilling all parts of his body.

25. Finally, take care of the environment. Switch off your phones, turn off the laptops, make sure there is no disturbance of any sort.

This movement is particularly relaxing. This erotic massage can help spice up your relationship at all levels. They will help, in any case, develop your complicity with your partner and allow you to pamper your love story.

CHAPTER 6. WHY SENSUALITY ENHANCES THE EXPERIENCE OF EROTIC MASSAGE

Erotic massage is first and foremost, a matter of atmosphere and sensuality. The more sensual an erotic massage is, the better you are going to enjoy it. Sensuality is marked by the appetite and passion of the body, a sexually exciting and gratifying experience. That is why you should not forget to lock the door, close the curtains, turn off the phones and beeps to avoid being disturbed in action. After that, take care of the massage area: preferably a bed or a massage table. Prepare towels to support the neck and knees. You can also use pillows, protected by a pillowcase clean and easy to wash. Spread a towel on the massage surface to avoid doing any stains with the massage oil. For an even more intimate and sensual atmosphere, plunging the room in the dim light. Avoid too strong lights.

Do not hesitate to cover the lamps with a thin sheet to create a romantic atmosphere, and light a few candles in the room. Arrange some incense sticks too, and turn them on. For those who do not wish to use incense, a refreshing spray can do the trick. Having fresh water near you is always welcome to hydrate yourself during the massage. Be sure to store your massage oil on the hand with extra towels to clean in case. Turn on the CD player with the CD ready for play. Finally, before starting the massage, I advise the two lovers to shower, cut their nails, and if necessary, shave.

Benefits of Erotic Massage for Couples' Relationship and Sex Life

The massage is a moment of relaxation that brings much well-being. This massage, which is called erotic, is a little different from others, but it is not about sex. The person who is massing will insist on the erogenous zones and practice soft and sensual touches in mutual respect.

It Helps One Relax

As with most massages, the goal is to relax areas of the body that are tense or slightly blocked. This allows you to revitalize your body if this is done regularly, you can also solve chronic muscle or tendon pain problems and improve your general health.

Erotic massage is also a perfect way to reactivate a good flow of energy in the body and balance the different points called chakras in the Indian and Chinese tradition. This is essential to feeling good about your body and achieving some form of inner balance, which is very important.

For the one who is massaged, the sensations are exquisite and can even sometimes lead to orgasm. However, this is not the goal, and the rules of the trade shows are strict.

Optimize and Improve the Functioning of the Relationship

Massage has been used in most cultures since ancient times for the benefits it brings to the body. Indeed, in addition to relaxation, it provides a multitude of positive aspects. In recent years, more and more scientists are studying its effects and showing us all that can be drawn from them.

Thus, some studies have shown that erotic massage is beneficial in most cases of joint pain because it relaxes the nerves and resorbs some swelling. It also contributes to the proper functioning of the cardiovascular system by promoting good blood circulation.

Other studies have shown that massage stimulates the immune system and reduces stress. It also helps regulate migraines and digestive pain. Thus, erotic massage is a great way to take care of your health, to treat specific pains, and to stay in shape. Also, many trade shows offer this type of services at affordable prices.

What are the benefits of the erotic massage for the body?

In a society where physical and mental strength is increasingly absorbed by the work and responsibilities of everyday life, "new diseases" harmful to humans have emerged, such as " burn-out ". This results in signs of exhaustion related to the arduousness of work — stress factor, insomnia, a permanent state of fatigue, up to depression.

What are the sources of well-being to dissolve these negative states toxic to our health? Breathing and relaxation techniques can help you reprogram. This is the case of relaxing massages and particularly sensual massage. It is important to see how and to determine what are the obvious benefits for everyone.

What happens to the Body During Erotic Massage?

By doing this type of massage, you will be surprised by the intense excitement of certain parts of your body, and through this, discover new erogenous zones that you did not suspect existed. An erotic massage must be a satisfying act for oneself (whether or not you reach orgasm). This is something that many couples appreciate, especially. It is a way and an opportunity for everyone to focus on giving, and the other to receive, and therefore not to give and receive simultaneously as it happens during coitus or other acts. It is a thoughtful and perfect way for the two members of the couple to get excited in any role and thus prolong intimacy.

The erotic massage is generally vital for women since it provides the same effect as that of a kiss, a caress, or other preliminary stakes. This effect can significantly increase the female sex hormones, responsible for the excitement and the preparation of her body to receive an orgasm.

The erotic or sensual massage also helps men with erection problems or prone to impotence. It may be that the first time, it takes a little time for the couple to relax. However, with a bit of practice, you can succeed in instilling massages with the intensity that will lead to very sensual experiences.

It is a perfect preamble in the search for orgasm and coitus - It serves to complement oneself, to find oneself in an unknown or forgotten universe and thus to get closer to one's partner - It is a sexual therapy in herself.

The erotic massage helps the treatment of premature ejaculation accompanied by other therapies adapted to this problem.

CHAPTER 7. TANTRIC AND LINGAM MASSAGE TIPS

Tantric massage, a dialogue of bodies to sublimate our sexuality, transcends our relationship, and unifies our relationship. Whether one is in low libido, in routine phase in the sexuality of our couple or search of new practices to resize our sex life, we all have good reasons to discover tantric massage.

Tantric is a massage designed to meet our quest for pleasure, to release our sexual energy while relaxing our mind. The tantric massage is a very sensual massage, and it aims to stimulate deeper sexual desires and libido. A tantric massage is a set of gentle caresses that are close to the sexual preliminaries between couples. Tantric massage is a loving prelude where a reunion with her body takes precedence. Much more than just a preliminary, this practice develops the art of harmonious relationship with one's partner. Touch, in the heart of the intimate!

How to do a tantric massage?

The course of a session is not technical and does not revolve around a specific gesture. Give and receive are the two poles. As for a dance, a real bodily dialogue between the two partners takes place. Each opens to the other. Slowness is required; it is often even the condition to "feel". Breathing is another central element in relaxing the mind. The idea would also be to find a thrill, a vibration source of profound well-being.

Sometimes, tremors occur, followed by a great relaxation, as if a cuirass flew away. The body can even become a temple, for a sexual relationship, where the sacred dimension is present.

Some tips for putting tantric massage into practice

Before you do a tantric massage, you need to take some steps:

Get rid of his day, to disconnect from the outside world; for example, you can take a shower to relax; you can spend time together, in silence. Before embarking on the massage, prepare this time together;

Create favorable conditions: an aromatic candle, a piece of music that you like, cushions, a massage oil...

Tantric massage: the key steps to getting started!

Tantric massage can be a prelude to lovemaking or restore a bodily dialogue and love between partners. Accessible to all, its benefits are many to start with sexuality, more conscious and fulfilled.

These are the key tips to getting started with a tantric massage;

Create A Sacred Space

Tantric massage requires a "sacred" space, that is to say, the intimacy between the two partners, for a deep connection with oneself, the other, and its spiritual dimension. To create such a space, it suffices to honor our five senses. Light a candle, symbol of the inner flame. Embellish the atmosphere with essential oil with recognized virtues to awaken sexuality. Put music that evokes love for you. Plan food and a drink for after (fruit and hot tea, or infusion with rose). On the floor, install several layers for comfort, a towel, and cushions around and fabrics of red, pink or orange, a color of passion.

Ask The Intention
The difference between wellness and tantric massage lies in the intention of the session. This practice proposes to restore a connection of our three centers; body, heart, mind, to allow a free circulation of the sexual energy or the vital energy. Sitting next to the person lying down, place the two joined hands in front of your heart, and state internally your intention to connect it to the energy of life.

Nudity, a Choice of Freedom
In Tantra, the most important thing is the respect of each person's freedom of being. The fact of being naked facilitates the fluidity of the movement. However, there is no obligation. Put yourself in the outfit where you will be comfortable to give up. Nudity is possible when it is lived in great freedom. It is up to everyone to decide.

The Quality of Presence

In a tantric massage, the quality of presence is essential. The masseur puts himself in an attitude of openness and hospitality. By opening yourself to the earth, sky connection, and emptying your thoughts, this is an attitude comparable to that of a meditator. The masseur will unambiguously awaken the natural sensuality of the body, source of our pleasure, but also our vitality. This practice appeals to your receptiveness and your ability to give up.

The Tantric Protocol

The proceedings of the massage are not based on a specific protocol. Giving and receiving are the two poles: as we see in a dance, a real body dialogue takes place between the two partners. However, if there is an instruction to be respected, it is the movement from bottom to top, the direction of flow of the sexual energy. Feet to the head, through the solar plexus. The massage takes place in the direction of the wave of the rise of orgasmic power, even if it is not an objective to reach absolutely.

Massage Slowly

Slowness is essential, and it is very often the condition to develop one's feelings. However, even more, it is the rhythm that is important, between slowness and fluidity faster. Playing with rhythm allows the mind of your partner to disconnect. Sometimes the hands stop to feel the energy flow. Sometimes they envelop the body in a wide movement. The breathing of both partners is another central element in practice.

The Good Movements

There are many movements in the practice of tantric massage. Significant smoothing, wrapping, fluttering, and many others. However, much more than a technique of movement, one must keep in mind to awaken the soul of the body, to re-circulate this sexual energy.

The Sex Massage

Tantric massage is not sexual, in the traditional sense of the word, that is to say, excitation, or stimulation of the erogenous zones. Sex, male or female, breasts, buttocks are included in the whole body. However, the intention is essential: it is to encompass and not to partition, nor to excite or stimulate, but to restore a sense of unity of the body. It is important for the person massed to specify if the massage is pleasant for him/her.

Professional Tantric Massage

A tantric massage that you receive in a professional setting must include specific quality criteria. A good practitioner must be clear about his intentions. There is no sexual connotation in this massage. If you do not feel respected, trust your feelings, and set your limits.

Tantric Massage: Physical and Relational Benefits

Tantric massage is not just relaxing, pleasure is the rendezvous, not sexual, but the body awakens to the senses. Be careful, and it is not a recipe to boost your libido; it is a relational commitment, an invitation to take care of others and oneself. Beyond the physical benefits, this practice also allows to "recover " your taste for love, sensuality, and sharing. It is also a way of letting go and a break to recognize your own needs. The relationship with your partner will take on a new sexual dimension, and gain in authenticity.

Tantric massage: Rediscover your partner

The tantric massage profoundly modifies the relational quality of the couple. Most of the time, the lack of desire or pleasure comes from the fact that one believes to know everything about the other, thus blocking any eventuality or any surprise on his part, including sexually. An area where perhaps more than elsewhere the routine threatens, with the mechanical aspect that we know.

This particular massage allows a rediscovery of the other, the quality of your partner's skin, his breath, curves, his sensuality. There is the idea of awakening, of going beyond what is believed of oneself and the other.

Lingam massage: what is it?

The lingam massage is a very sensual massage. This massage is a tantric massage recommended for men with erectile dysfunction, those who are severely lacking self-confidence and those who want to learn more about their body.

So why this name may seem weird?
The lingam is the Sanskrit name for the sex of the man. It also translates as "Wand of Light". Tantrism is known to treat sexuality in a sacred way, and lingam is always honored with respect.

A lingam massage is a part of the tantric massage. This is where the masseuse will massage with specific gestures lingam, perineum, testicles, or the sacred point (small groove between the testicles and anus).

The purpose of a lingam massage is not to lead to orgasm but to learn to control your body and discover new sensations. It will teach you to reclaim your body, to regain confidence in you, and to relax.

These are the key tips to getting started with a lingam massage;

You will be in a room where everything will be done for you to relax. You will lie on your back and of course naked.

Your partner will gently massage every part of your body to relax. She will then pour a little oil on the body of the lingam and the testicles.

You will start by massaging the testicles, then the body of the lingam and finally his head.

As she looks after you, you will feel more and more relaxed. You will explore new sensations, and you will learn to receive this gentle and sensual massage.

CHAPTER 8. TOP 10 EROGENOUS ZONES ON WOMEN AND MEN

Are you sure you know all the X rated areas of male and female pleasure? Have you ever heard of point P? Discover the top 10 erogenous zones in humans. Some areas of the body that we do not always think about are particularly sensitive to caresses.

This classification of the male erogenous zones is based on a scientific study, in which men were asked to rate out of ten the intensity of the sexual arousal that gave them contact with different areas of their body. Each partner has its specificities, it is, however, essential to probe your man to know if, yes or no, this or that zone is well erogenous at home. (Read more on the study here https://www.ncbi.nlm.nih.gov/m/pubmed/239932 82/)

Firstly, let us consider the men;

The glans and the brake

The glans, located at the end of the penis, is circled by a bead called the "crown". If the sex of the man remains the most erogenous zone, the glans is one of the body parts richest in sensory sensors and therefore, the most reactive to pleasure. To make your partner shudder, firmly grasp the base of her sex, lean towards her glans, and lick it gently.

If they are the most sensitive areas of the male body (its female counterparts would be the clitoris and its edge), they are also the most sensitive: they require special care while being very delicate. Do not approach too eagerly, and not to squat too long, especially. Finally, it is essential that these intimate and fragile parts are always well lubricated. Otherwise, it could irritate your other half.

The rod

The other vast ranked X region of the male anatomy is the body of the penis. Although very sensitive, the penis suffers less contact, and you can, therefore, pamper it more.

The Mouth

Oh yes! Although this area is relatively overused, it has lost nothing of its beauty. Thus, it appears as one of the top zones of excitement, for both men and women. Moreover, it is true that a kiss with the tongue between wet lips, it does its little effect!

The testicles

Family jewels are to be treated with care too. The most delicate attentions will be the best received. Avoid the nails, teeth, suctions, and other stimulations too strong in these places. The slogans are delicacy and finesse.

Neck

This part is quite prone to chills. It is simple and often kisses on the neck is very useful,

The nipples

Licking the nipples of boys is not an aberration, no, evidenced by the excitement caused by sharp licks on them.

The perineum

This area between the anus and the beginning of the testicles is no more favorable to feverishness. Indeed, this point can be stimulated with more tonicity than the rest of the penis, but also, it encourages orgasm. In short: an appointment not to be missed!

The anus

This is one of the weirdest erogenous zones in men. Moreover, yet, stimulating the anus by introducing a finger can be particularly exciting. Go slowly and watch his reaction.

Ears

A little cliché perhaps and certainly not to everyone's taste, for some, the ears have magical powers (on erection).

The point P or the prostate

To approach with many precautions! It is in the anus that we find this erogenous zone the size of a small apricot. Although the P-point is very rich in nerve endings and can cause much excitement, many men are reluctant to be touched at this point. Ditto for the buttocks that are, symbolically and physically, very related to anal pleasure.

Moreover, even...

The crotch, lower abdomen, and groin are very closely connected sensory areas, sex, and caresses on these regions inevitably generate the revival! Precisely like the inside of the thighs, which is an area that is too often neglected even though many men like to be caressed and touched there.

Of course, as rightly pointed out by one of the men I interviewed, the most erogenous zone for every human being is the heart: "With my girlfriend, they are everywhere... Basically: our complicity associated with love makes my whole body erogenous... Even when it touches my knee, I am excited".

Let us now consider women. Women are much more sensitive and full of different places!

Clitoris

The clitoris and its edge are the most sensitive part of a woman, and they require special care while being very delicate. Just like the male glans, you do not approach the clitoris too eagerly, and you handle this part with care in other not to irritate your partner.

Buttocks

The buttocks, in women as in men, contain many nerve endings. Their supple texture makes them a fascinating erotic adventure playground that lends itself to many forms of stimulation, as they can offer different sensations. The buttocks can be stimulated by pinching or gently biting them. You can also caress the fold between the buttock and the thigh, a sensitive area, with your fingertips.

Armpits

The armpits are also an erogenous zone that we neglect too often. Moreover, yet, they can give much pleasure to your partner. The skin is fragile at this point, which makes them particularly sensitive to petting. But be careful not to tickle her, the goal being to make her crazy, not to make her laugh.

Neck

On the nape of the neck, the skin is most often devoid of adipose tissue, which increases the sensations provided by caresses and kisses.

Nipples

The nipples (the nipples and the colored part that surrounds them) are an area of the chest apart. Their hypersensitivity requires subtle and meticulous caresses, but they promise pleasant sensations.

The ear

You certainly know, women love to be whispered naughty little words in the hollow of the ear before the antics. Sensitive, this area awakens the sexual desire of women and allows to increase the excitement gradually. The lobe of the ear is particularly vulnerable to kisses and small nibbling.

Inside thighs

Stimulating the inside of the legs is like turning around the bush. It is a source of pleasure that intensifies as we get closer to his crotch.

Mouth

The mouth just as in men is also one of the top erogenous zones in women.

Foot

This is another erogenous zone that is neglected by many people. When handled well, a good erotic massage on foot excites women a lot.

Breast

Men love this part, and it excites women a lot too.

The lower belly

Before reaching the most specific area, the lower belly is also very receptive to caresses of all kinds.

The Vagina

Yes, this is also a very sensitive part of a woman.

Let us look at the degree of excitements on these areas on a scale of 10.

For women

1. The clitoris (Note: 9.1 / 10. Is it not, ladies?)

2. The vagina (8.4, yes, everything is connected)

3. The mouth and the lips (7.9 This is why we love so many kisses.)

4. The top of the neck (7.5 so sensual)

5. Breasts (7.3, even if they are small! -It is not the size that counts)

6. The nipples (7.3 This is not a reason to bite them thoroughly, huh!)

7. Inside thighs (6,7)

8. Nape (6.2 with vampire kisses)

9. The ears (5. Big debate.)

10. The lower back (4,7).

For men

1. The penis (note: 9/10)

2. The mouth and the lips (note: 7. So, if we kissed even more?)

3. The testicles (6.5)

4. Inside thighs (5,8)

5. The top of the neck (5.6 Roar!)

6. The nipples (4.89, Attention, the subject is sensitive)

7. The pubis (4,81)

8. The perineum (4.80)

9. The neck (4,5)

10. The ears (4,3).

In short, we have lots of erogenous zones that are very intense and pleasurable. You only need to discover these zones in your partner.

As everyone knows, it would be wrong to reduce personal enjoyment to the only these parts; the nipples, buttocks, anus, and many others. The whole body is a real playground, a sensation piano on which you can tap all the keys. To always provide more pleasure to your partner, explore his/her body, know his/her most sensitive areas, and exploit them to propel him/her straight to the seventh heaven.

CHAPTER 9. BEST MASSAGE POINTS FOR SEDUCTION, RELAXATION, AND SEX

These valuable points are chosen for their ability to calm a person down, making the preliminaries more sensitive and considerate, and sex more exciting. It is important to be caring and gentle and gently rub or massage these points with love, like a soft kiss, and no harsh pressure. In general, I advise creating a quiet space for you and your partner. Almost all excitement problems are psychological, not physical. Since our society today praises agitation and stress, our bodies and minds never have time to be bored. However, boredom is essential to our human existence.

This is the basis on which any increase in the actual libido can occur, as opposed to the artificial increase of drugs or pornography. By forcing boredom on the body, people will settle into a more relaxed state so that they are mentally and physically available for intimacy.

Everyone and all bodies are different, and the most important aspects of improving your sex life come from within. Communication, trust, and relaxation are the keys. Besides, there is still not enough scientific research on the pleasure of sex, and there is no golden standard for doing it. These pressure points help to increase calm and reduce stress, which can increase pleasure and communication during sex. It is not recommended to use these points only for sexual pleasure.

Here are the best massage points for seduction, relaxation, and sex;

Head massage

To know how to massage the head, your partner must be lying on the back, comfortably. He/she must be able to relax completely and feel no discomfort. You will start by putting both hands on his forehead by touching it.

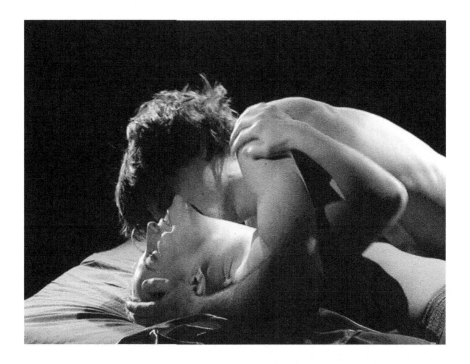

Start from the nose to go up to the top of his forehead, to his hair. Pass your right hand then your left hand and so on. Slowly, slowly, while varying the pressure of your actions according to the pleasure of your partner. Do this 10 to 15 times then position the palms of your hands on his temples, staying about 2 minutes.

You can also massage his scalp. For this, make circular movements as if you were shampooing, but with delicacy and sensuality.

By doing this massage, you will allow your partner to relax and feel light. There is an energy center behind the front. Do not forget the ears! They are very sensitive and erogenous zones. However, some people do not like being ventured to their ears so test before going too far.

Back massage

To know how to massage the back, your partner must be lying on the belly. As for you, you must place yourself at the level of his head. You will put your hands flat on the top of his back. Then your palms will have to slide slowly to the buttocks.

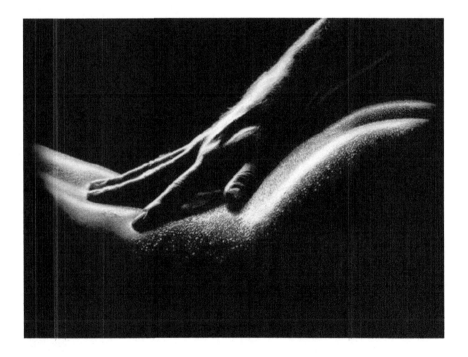

Make a pressure move at the roundness of his/her buttocks, slide on her flanks, and go up to her armpits. Finally, gently pull your shoulders up to start the process again. Adapt the pressure according to the desires of your partner.

Also, think about adapting your gestures according to the breathing of your partner. Go down in the expiry phase and go back to the inspiration phase.

Breast massage

To massage the breast of your partner, turn to her right at the height of her hips. You will place your hands on her chest. A hand on her pectoral/left breast and a hand on her pectoral/right breast.

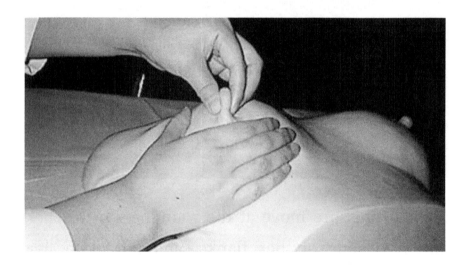

You will make circular inverted movements, i.e., clockwise for the right side and in the opposite direction for the left side. Do this simultaneously, taking care to wrap the breastplate/breast tightly with your entire hand.

You can take the opportunity to add kisses and licks on the nipples but always stay in the sensuality and delicacy.

Arms massage

To massage the arms of your partner, sit next to him. The latter is still lying down. Take his left hand in your right hand and place your left hand on his wrist with your fingers toward his shoulder.

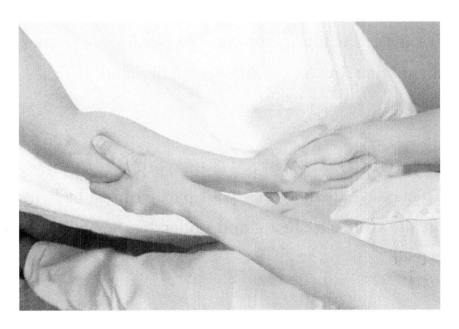

Move your left hand from his wrist to his elbow and continue to his shoulder before lowering his entire arm and starting again. Afterward, use both hands synchronously, side by side, to climb from his forearm to his shoulder by adjusting the pressure.

To go back down, keep both hands in sync but do less downward pressure. Then take his hand in yours and knead his palm using your thumbs. Finally, slide the fingers of your hand between his fingers, palm against palm, and make a few circles to the right and to the left to relax his wrists.

Do these movements several times for the other arm. For the erotic touch, you can kiss her fingers or suck them, one by one, with sensuality and delicacy, always.

Buttocks massage

To massage the buttocks, your partner must be lying on the stomach. Just stand under his/her buttocks astride.

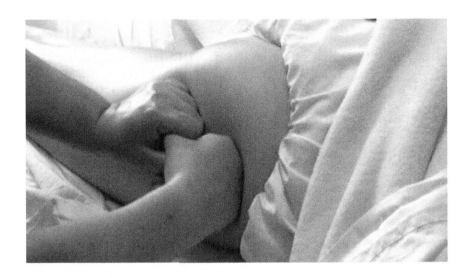

Use the palms of your hands to make circular movements on the buttocks simultaneously. Increase the pressure little by a little while listening to your partner. (You can also use your forearms for more pressure and more significant movements.)

Then concentrate on the right buttock and then on the left buttock. For each of the buttocks, you will use your thumbs to make a wave of skin and up to the coccyx.

Remember that the buttocks love the pressure, so do yourself and enjoy it more vigorously in this area.

Foot massage

These are considered strong points for balancing the subtle energies in the body while simultaneously promoting an increase in blood flow to the heart of the body.

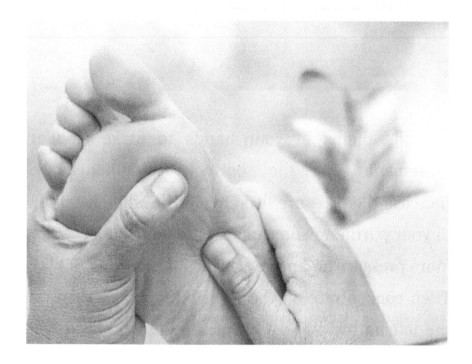

CHAPTER 10. TYPES OF MASSAGE TO TRY ON YOUR PARTNER

Look into your partner's eyes when you start touching his genitals. Make sure that the connection you made at the beginning of the massage still exists; if it does not, try to restore it by slowing down and asking your partner some questions about what he or she is experiencing. When continuing the genital massage, remember to use your free hand to tease the rest of your partner's body.

Female genital massage

Start by gently rubbing the entire vulva, following with clitoral stimulation, and finishing with internal and clitoral stimulation - do not forget the G-spot! Vaginal penetration can only take place in case of a fairly extreme level of awakening. If your partner is comfortable, feel free to use a vibrator to help you with the massage.

Male genital massage

Begin by applying a lubricant into the palm of your hands and gently applying it to the penis and testicles. Male genital massage is guided by one essential principle: to slow down and stop or change what you are doing just before ejaculation becomes inevitable. Keep him on the verge of ejaculation as much as possible. Ask your partner to let you know if he is about to ejaculate, which may have the effect of making him enjoy immediately if he is too excited or develops a signal - Change the pace. Play with the brake, caress him, and tickle him.

The massage is nearing completion. By bringing your partner to the extreme limit without allowing him to ejaculate, you prolong the massage and help him to have a more intense orgasm, powerful, if he wishes it.

Sensual or erotic massages

Sensual massage, erotic massage, body-body, and sexual massage are relaxing massages but can go beyond relaxation and well-being. This massage is very different from a traditional massage.

It involves good communication with the other, in a mutual spirit of trust and abandonment. It is sensual in the sense that the gestures are more caresses with a strong erotic tendency. These caresses are worn all over the body, including - but not only - on the genital and intimate parts, for the pleasure and enjoyment of the person who receives them.

This massage is very gradual to appreciate the continuous rise of pleasure better, and intermediate levels are established to slow down and enjoy more of the moment and increase desire.

The pleasure of the person being massaged is the main objective of this massage which can enter the game of caresses not only with the hand, the fingers but also the lips, the tongue, tissues or any other thing contributing to this excitement.

Because some people need to feel the desire of the other to feel theirs better and to express it better, the masseur will let himself be wholly undressed or even suggest to continue with a body-body massage.

Also, some people wishing to go further penetrations will accept the use of their stimulators, their intimate toys or the active participation of the masseur, his fingers, his tongue, his hooded sex, then leading to sex massage.

Body to body massage

This massage is exceptional. It is incredibly erotic and supposes the active participation of the two people who become in turn part of the massage of the other. It is practiced naked, body to body. The body of each is put to contribution, and it is not only hands that massage but the whole body, from head to toe. It implies a willingness to give as much as to receive.

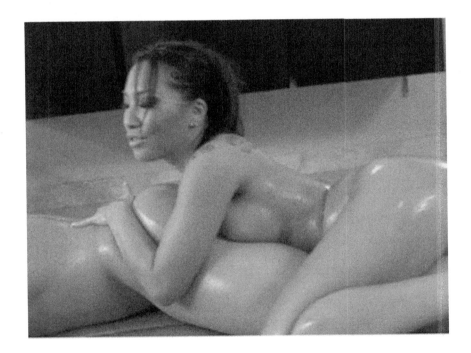

Although the genitals are thus laid bare, it is not a matter of making banal sexual intercourse. On the contrary, the intensity of this massage is stronger when the couples agree to practice it without sexual penetration despite the natural and visible excitement of the moment. This does not prevent the two people involved in this massage to feel desire, or even to enjoy intensely.

In conclusion, on a table nearby, have sweets: fresh fruit, chocolates, and why not champagne in an ice bucket? Choose soft music that invites you to tenderness. If you like the smell, burn incense.

Printed in Great Britain
by Amazon